YOUR KNOWLEDGE HAS VALUE

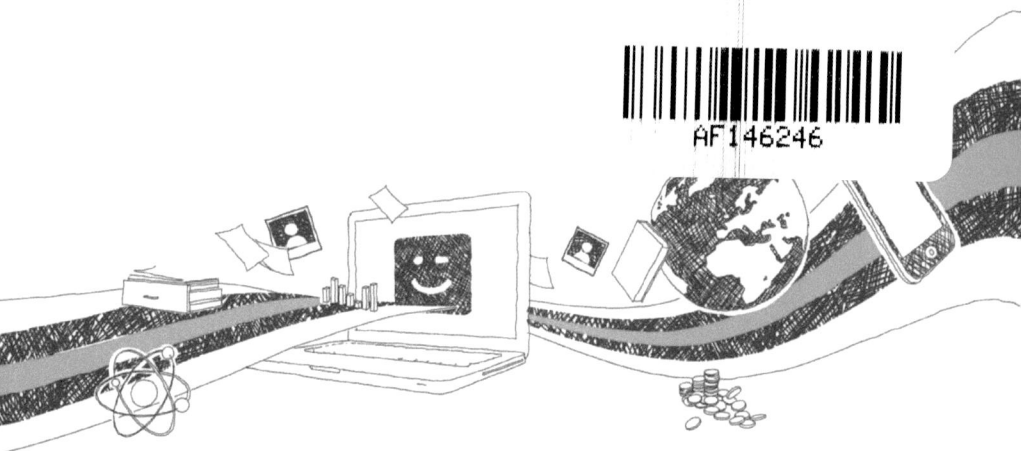
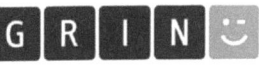

Bibliographic information published by the German National Library:

The German National Library lists this publication in the National Bibliography; detailed bibliographic data are available on the Internet at http://dnb.dnb.de .

Imprint:

Copyright © 2015 GRIN Verlag, Open Publishing GmbH
Print and binding: Books on Demand GmbH, Norderstedt Germany
ISBN: 978-3-668-11434-0

This book at GRIN:

http://www.grin.com/en/e-book/312457/a-preliminary-study-on-urinary-bladder-lesions-of-cattle-slaughtered-at

Jaleta Shuka Gurumu

A Preliminary Study On Urinary Bladder Lesions Of Cattle Slaughtered At Hashim Export Abattoir, Debrzeit

GRIN Publishing

GRIN - Your knowledge has value

Since its foundation in 1998, GRIN has specialized in publishing academic texts by students, college teachers and other academics as e-book and printed book. The website www.grin.com is an ideal platform for presenting term papers, final papers, scientific essays, dissertations and specialist books.

Visit us on the internet:

http://www.grin.com/

http://www.facebook.com/grincom

http://www.twitter.com/grin_com

ADDIS ABABA UNIVERSITY COLLEGE OF VETERINARY MEDICINE AND AGRICULTURE

A PRELIMINARY STUDY ON URINARY BLADDER LESSIONS OF CATTLE SLAUTHERED AT ONE OF RECOGNIZED EXPORT ABATTOIR DEBRZEIT, ETHIOPIA.

BY

JALETA SHUKA GURUMU

DVM thesis

December 2015

Debre Zeit, Ethiopia

TABLE OF CONTENTS   Page

TABLE OF CONTENTS i

LIST OF TABLES ii

LIST OF FIGURE iii

LIST OF ABBREVIATIONS iv

ACKNOWLEDGEMENTS v

1. INTRODUCTION 1

2. MATERIALS AND METHODS 4

2.1 Study area 4

2.2 Study animals 5

2.3 Sampling method 5

2.4 Ante mortem examination 6

2.5 Gross examination and characterization of urinary bladder lesions 6

2.6 Data analysis 7

3. RESULT 8

3.1. Prevalence of urinary bladder lesion 8

3.2. Risk factors and urinary bladder lesion 9

3.2.1. Breed and urinary bladder lesion 9

3.2.2. Body condition and urinary bladder lesion 9

3.2.3. Age and urinary bladder lesion 10

3.3. Prevalence of urinary bladder lesion by breed, age categories and body condition 11

3.4. Histopathological finding 11

4. DISCUSION 15

5. CONCLUSION AND RECOMMENDATIONS 16

6. REFERENCES 17

7. ANNEX 20

LIST OF TABLES

Table 1.The occurrence and types of urinary bladder lesions detected in male cattle slaughtered at Debre Zeit Elfora abattoir 8

Table 2. The prevalence of urinary bladder lesion by breed..9

Table 3. The prevalence of urinary bladder lesion by body condition............................10

Table 4. The prevalence of urinary bladder lesion age categories.................................10

Table 5. Risk factors associated with the occurrence of urinary bladder lesions...............11

Table 6. Distribution of Cases according to Microscopic Diagnosis..............................12

LIST OF FIGURE Pages

Figure -1. Map of the study area...4

Figure -2: Chronic non-specific cystitis with lymphoid aggregates in lamina propria 13

Figure -3: Chronic non-specific cystitis with lymphoid aggregates in lamina propria............13

Figure -4: Papillary urothelial neoplasm of low malignant potential 14

Figure -5 - Low grade papillary urothelial carcinoma showing papillae with mild pleomorphism cells with maintained basal polarity...14.

LIST OF ABBREVIATIONS

AAU	Addis Ababa University
BEH	Bovine enzootic hematuria
BPV	Bovine papiloma virus
CSA	Central Statistical Agency
CVMA	College of Veterinary Medicine
^0C	Degree Celsius
DVM	Doctor of Veterinary Medicine
FVM	Faculty of Veterinary Medicine
IBVP	Inactivated Bacterial Vaccine Production
EEA	Elfora Export Abattoir
Km	kilometer
Mm	Millimeter
PLC	Private Limited Company
SPP	Species
SPSS	Statistical Package for the Social Sciences
UTI	urinary tract infection

ACKNOWLEDGMENT

First and most, I would like to express my heartfelt thanks to God, for his everlasting love up on me. Secondly, I would like to express my deep gratitude to my co-Adivisor Mr. Hika Waktole for cooperation, constructive suggestions and encouragement during my research work. I am extremely thankful to all staff of National Veterinary Institute; particularly to personnel of IBVP section for their unreserved cooperation for the success of my career thought my study period. Thanks also to all workers of this abbaitor, for their cooperation during abattoir work. My deepest gratitude goes to Dr. Berecha Bayessa for his overall gudice, devotion of his precious time to correct this thesis paper. Last but not least, my appreciation goes to my family for love, support and encouragement.

ABSTRACT

The study was conducted from December 2014 to April 2015 aimed to determine the prevalence and types of urinary bladder lesions of local and exotic breeds of male cattle slaughtered at one of the recognized Debre Zeit abattoir. The urinary bladders of 325 male cattle were removed, inspected and opened to detect gross lesions. The prevalence of urinary bladder lesions was found to be 6.5% (21/325). Chronic cystitis was the most frequent finding and account 66.7% (14/21) of the total urinary bladder lesions, while acute cystitis was verified in 33.3% (7/21) of the cases. Regarding to the breeds, the prevalence of 6.1% (18/297) and 10.7% (3/28) were found in local and exotic, respectively. Out of 21urinary bladder lesions, 14 cases were diagnosed as chronic cystitis while 7 cases were acute cystitis. The lesions of chronic cystitis were variable and categorized as uncomplicated, proliferative, hypertrophied, dilated, and emphysematous and that of acute cystitis were hemorrhagic and purulent. Regarding histological examination point of view from the total 21 cases inflammatory lesions were (14%) while carcinoma was present in (86%) patients The occurrence of urinary bladder lesion was not statistical association with breed, age categories and body condition (p>0.05,) of the animal. Finally, conclusive remarks and recommendations on future areas of research are forwarded.

Key Words: *Abattoir, Cystitis, Cattle, Debre Zeit, Urinary Bladder.*

1. INTRODUCTION

The urinary bladder maybe involved with descending or ascending infections of the urinary system or uroliiasis that may result in obstruction of urine outlet with subsequent rapture and infiltration of urine to adjacent tissue (Blood and Radositis, 1994).

Lower urinary tract problems, in general the urinary bladder in particular are usually sporadic in occurrence (Ordonez and Rosia, 1996). Disorders of the urinary bladder are relatively uncommon and various types of etiological factors can affect the urinary bladder of bovine species. Inflammation of the lower urinary tract revolves around inflammation of the bladder. Under normal circumstances, the bladder is resistant to infection and bacteria are quickly eliminated by the normal flow of normal urine. Predisposition to urinary tract infection (UTI) occurs when there is stagnation of urine due to obstruction, incomplete voiding at micturation, or urothelial trauma, normal voiding is not sufficient to prevent and eliminate bladder infection. Incomplete voiding at micturation may be a result of diverticula of the urinary bladder or vesicoureteral reflux. The presence of residual urine can maintain a bladder infection allowing organisms to take advantage of any opportunity to invade the urothelium. The usual causes of cystitis are bacteria from the urethra, which are almost always from the rectal flora. A variety of bacteria may be involved in bladder infections such as: *Escherichia coli, proteus vulgaris*, sterptococcus and staphylococcus species are common pathogens that may cause cystitis in many species of animals, corynebacterium renal is important in cow (Blood and Radositis, 1994).

Caliculi may form in any part of the urinary duct system from the renal pelvis to the urethra but, urolithasis can cause obstructive lesions in the lower urinary tract and is known to cause significant problems in cattle. Obstructive urolithasi is almost exclusively a disease in males and primarily

1

affect steers. Urethral obstruction has been found to be one of the dominant surgical problems of oxen in and around Debre Zeit (Roman, 2000). Calculi in the urinary bladder are usually accompanied by a varying degree of chronic cystitis (Blood and Radositis, 1994).Cystitis may also develop secondary to congenital anomalies (Ehnen, 1990). Developmental abnormalities, hyperplasia and neplasia could also be involved in causing urinary bladder lesions (Herenda *et al.*, 1990).

Enzootic hematuria of cattle is severing syndrome caused by prolonged ingestion of toxic principles of bracken fern (peteridium species). Urinary bladder tumors associated with this syndrome are common in 4 to 12 year old cattle urinary bladder. Neoplasms are common only in cattle where they are associated with bracken fern or related ferns (Pamuckal *et al.*, 1976, Muckenzie, 1978, Rao *et al.*, 1990; Campo *et al.*, 1992, Sardon et al., 2005). Recent studies demonstrate a strong relationship between papillomaviruses and some clastogenic, mutagenic and/or carcinogenic principles of bracken fern. DNA of bovine papilloma virus type 2 (BPV-2) was found in 69% of experimental and in 46% of naturally occurring bladder cancers. The high degree of association between bladder cancers and BPV-2 suggests that this virus plays role in bladder oncogenesis. This plant causes different pathological symptoms mainly because it contains two different toxic principles one radio mimetic carcinogenic compound, the norsesqui terpenc ptaquiloside (Hirono *et al.*, 1984) and a thiaminase principle is the one which cause bovine enzootic hematuria(BEH) (Heeschen, 1959, Rosenberger and Heeschen 1960; Rosenberger 1965, Dobereiner *et al.*, 1967). The nature of the bladder tumors, associated with the ingestion of bracken fern, is quite peculiar. Epithelial tumors as well as mesenchymal tumors have been described besides the strange capacity to induce different neoplasms in same animals(Jokarnia *et al.*, 2000).

Parasitic infections of the urinary system are not of major importance in domestic animals. The urinary form of schistosomiasis in domestic animals appears to occur only in cattle heavily infected with *schistosoma mattheei* a parasite of the mesentric and hepatic portal veins of ruminants. The lesions in the urinary bladder may range fromscattered individual granuloms with petechia to wide spread polypoid granular patches(Jones *et al.*, 1997).

Diseases of the urinary system are of considerable importance in many cattle raising countries. Problems associated with the urinary bladder can cause significant loss in the live stock industry particularly when they are complicated with obstructive lesions. Very few studies have been conducted in Ethiopia in regard to disorders of the urinary tract.

Thus, the objective of study is:

❖ To determine the prevalence of gross and histological urinary bladder lesions on adult cattle slaughtered at one of recognized Debre Zeit Export Abattoir.

2. MATERIALS AND METHODS

2.1. Study area

The study was conducted on Bishoftu town, from October 2013 to May 2014. Bishoftu is located 47km south east of Addis Ababa. The area is located at 9^0N latitude and 40^0E longitudes at an altitude of 1850 meters above sea level in central high land of Ethiopia. The town has an annual rainfall of 866 mm of which 84% is in the long rainy season (June to September). The dry season extends from October to February. The mean annual maximum and minimum temperatures are 26^0c and 14^0c respectively humidity of 61.3% (CSA, 2003).

Figure 1. Map of the study area

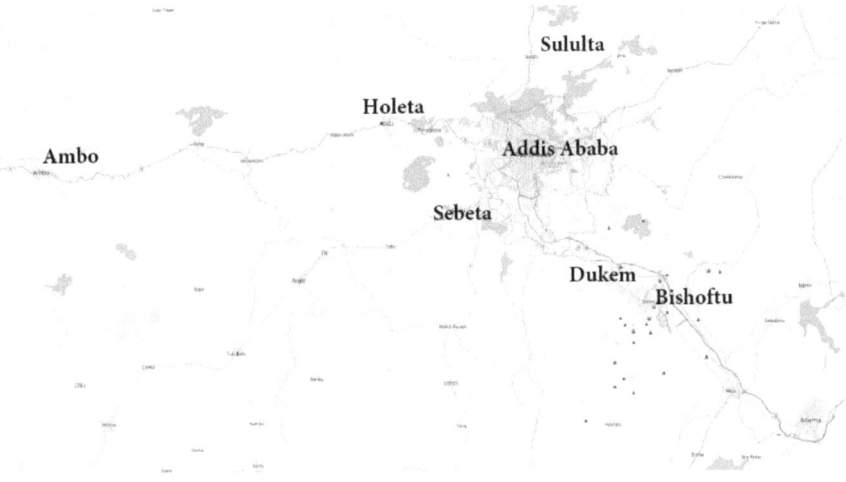

Source: http://www.openstreetmap.org/#map=9/9.1157/38.4947 , edited.

Suburb communities of Bishoftu town use a mixed crop and livestock farming system. These communities are shifting their livelihood for agriculture since land has been occupied by industries. The town is one of the growing industrial towns of the country due to proximity to capital city and accessibility for all types of transportation mean. This Abattoir PLC is the one companies established in Bishoftu for export sheep and goat meat to the Middle East countries.

2.2. Study Animals and design

Local and Exotic cattle breed originated from Awassa, Borena, Shashemane, Arsi-Bale, Somali lowland areas and from northern Shoa highland were used. All these animals from different origin where kept under extensive production system. The animals were transported long distance by tracks kept at the lairage for two up to three days waiting slaughter without sufficient feed and water.

2.3. Sampling method

Total of 38 conventional visits were made to examine urinary bladder samples at the export abattoir. An average of 30 head of cattle was slaughtered five days per week. Only male cattle of different age groups were included. Conventional sampling method was employed to examine the desired number of cattle. During the course of study, urinary bladders from 325 cattle were collected for examination. Clinical and gross positive finding samples were sent to laboratory for histopathological examination. The material for the study was comprised of biopsy from transurethral resection of bladder Tissue (TURBT)

Inclusion Criteria

All the TURBT biopsies received in the department of Pathology, College Of Veterinary Medicine and Agriculture

Exclusion Criteria

- Autolysed specimen

- Inadequate biopsies.

Biopsy specimens were processed as per routine histopathological technique. Paraffin section was cut and stained by haematoxylin and eosin. Then bladder lesions were studied according to ISUP (2004) classification (Annex 2)

2.4.Antimortun examination

The ante mortem examination was under taken to score the body condition of study animals. The description given by Delahunta and Hable (1986) (Annex 1) was used to estimate the ages of the animals. The animals were inspected before they were slaughtered for body condition scored as fat, medium and lean following the description given by Nicholson and Butterworth (1986) (Annex1)

2.5.Gross examination and characterization of urinary bladder lesions

The urinary bladders where removed at its neck and a more detail examination was carried out after the urine has been discarded. First post mortem examination was made by visual inspection and then palpation was done on the specific organ for the presence of any lesion. The gross appreance, consistency and size of the lesion were considered to state the pathological lesion. The examinations were started with serosal surface of the urinary bladders followed by systematic opening of the urinary bladder. After incision of the bladders   mucosae were inspected very carefully for the presence of any abnormalities.

Gross description of cystitis was conducted by considering the description of Herenda *et al.,* (1990). The pathological lesions were generally classified in to acute and chronic cystitis. The bladders were diagnosed as acute cystitis when the mucosa of urinary bladder was hyperemic but not thickened. On the other hand, urinary bladders with redness thickened mucosa were considered as chronic cystitis. The acute lesions were further classified as hemorrhagic and purulent according the presence bleeding and involvement of secondary infection, respectively. However, the chronically infected urinary bladder were grouped in to uncomplicated, proliferative, dilated, hypertrophied and emphysematous (Herenda *et al.,* 1990). The bladders with nodular, villous, papillary projections or extensive corrugation were as proliferative chronic cystitis while bladders with rough coarsely granular or irregular reddened and thickened mucosa with no proliferative lesion are classified as uncomplicated chronic cystitis. Enlarged urinary bladder without thickened wall and almost transparent were said to be dilated and enlarged bladders with thickened wall was taken as hypertrophied urinary bladders (Shimeles, 2008 and Ayalew, 2002).

2.6. Data analysis

The collected data during sampling was entered and stored into Microsoft Office Excel spread sheet 2007. The data were thoroughly screened before subjecting to statistical analysis. Descriptive statistics was used for data presentation. The study variables were analyzed using computer software SPSS (version 20.0). Categorical variables were analyzed using chi-square. The statistical significance of the study variables were evaluated at $p < 0.05$.

3. RESULT

3.1. Prevalence of urinary bladder lesion

The prevalence of urinary bladder lesion in male local and exotic cattle breed slaughtered at this Abattoir was found to be 6.5% (21/325) (tab.1). Gross examination of the lesions revealed that 4.3% (n=14) was diagnosed as chronic while 2.2% (n=7) was acute cystitis (tab.1). The higher chronic cystitis (5 cases) was uncomplicated lesions followed by 3 cases of proliferative lesion. The rest chronic lesions were identified as dilation, hypertrophic, and emphysematous with two cases each. On the other hand, those of eight acute cystitis bladders were identified as hemorrhagic (5 cases) and purulent (3 cases) (Tab.1).

Table 1. The occurrence and types of urinary bladder lesions detected in male cattle slaughtered at Debre Zeit Elfora abattoir

Cystitis type	No. of animals	Percentage (%)
Acute	**7**	**33.3**
Haemorrhagic	5	
Purulent	2	
Chronic	**14**	**66.7**
Uncomplicated	5	
Proliferative	3	
Dilated	1	
Hypertrophy	1	
Emphysematous	4	
Total	**21**	**100**

3.2. Risk factors of urinary bladder lesion

3.2.1. Breed and urinary bladder lesions

The breed wise distribution of urinary bladder lesion higher prevalence of 10.7% (3/28) was recorded in exotic breed slaughtered at this Export Abattoir as compare to 6.1% (18/297) prevalence of lesion in local breed (tab. 2). However, there is no statistical significant (p>0.05) difference between the two breed.

Table 2. The prevalence of urinary bladder lesion by breed

Risk factors	No. of animals examined	No. of animals with lesions	Percentage
Breed			
Local	297	18	6.1
Exotic	28	3	10.7

3.2.2. Body condition and urinary bladder lesions

Comparatively similar urinary bladder lesion prevalence of 6.4% (n=5), 5.6 % (n=10) and 8.8 % (n=6) were observed in cattle having fatty, moderate and lean body condition, respectively (Table 3). The respective urinary bladder lesion in different body condition having cattle was not found to be significant.

Table 3. The prevalence of urinary bladder lesion by body condition

Risk factors	No. of animals examined	No. of animals with lesions	Percentage
Body condition			
Moderate	179	10	5.6
Lean	68	6	8.8
Fatty	78	5	6.4

3.2.3. Age and urinary bladder lesions

The age ranges of animals examined in this study were 4 to 12 years. Cattle with age ranges of 4-7 years (7.1%) were more involved with urinary bladder lesions when compared with others age categories (5.6%) (Table 4). However the difference was not statistically significant (P> 0.05).

Table 4. The prevalence of urinary bladder lesion age categories

Risk factors	No. of animals examined	No. of animals with lesions	Percentage
Age categories			
4-7	183	13	7.1
8-12	142	8	5.6

10

3.3. Prevalence of urinary bladder lesion by breed, age categories and body condition

The test statistic showed no statistically significant between the risk factors and the occurrence of urinary bladder lesions (p>0.05) (Table 5).

Table 5. Risk factors associated with the occurrence of urinary bladder lesions. Where (L=Local, E=Exotic) and (F= Fat, M=Moderate, L=Lean).

Lesions	Breed		Age		Body Condition		
	L	E	4-7	8-12	F	M	L
Present	18	3	13	8	5	10	6
Absent	279	25	169	135	76	16	860
Chi-square	0.338		0.615		0.855		
P-value	0.917		0.433		0.652		

3.4. Histophatolocal finding

Total of 21 TURBT biopsies were analyzed. A spectrum of different pathological lesions was observed in the study. In this study most common age group was 8-12 years of urinary bladder lesions where more detected by histopathological examination. In the present study, total cases of inflammatory lesions were (14%) while carcinoma was present in (86%) patients. The most common microscopic diagnosis was high-grade papillary urothelial carcinoma (38.5%) while the least common microscopic diagnosis was moderately differentiate adenocarcinoma and eosinophilic cystitis (5%) and other microscopic diagnosis were also found like low-grade papillary urothelial carcinoma (23%) Papillary urothelial neoplasm of low malignant potential (9.5%) chronic non-specific cystitis (9.5%) moderately differentiated squamous cell carcinoma (9.5%) (Figure – 2, 3, 4,) (Table 6)

11

Table 6. Distribution of Cases according to Microscopic Diagnosis

Microscopic Diagnosis	No.	%
Inflammatory Lesions	**3**	**14**
Chronic non-specific cystitis	2	9.5
Eosinophilic cystitis	1	5
Carcinoma	**18**	**86**
High-grade papillary urothelial carcinoma	8	38.5
Low-grade papillary urothelial carcinoma	5	23
Moderately differentiated adeno carcinoma	1	5
Moderately differentiated squamous cell carcinoma	2	9.5
Papillary urothelial neoplasm of low malignant potential	2	9.5
Total	**21**	**100**

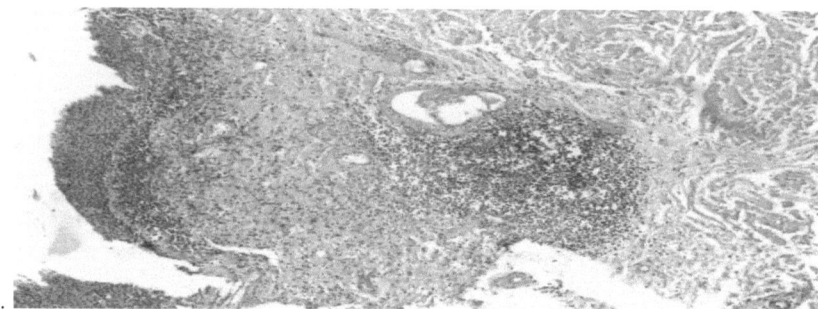

Figure -2: Chronic non-specific cystitis with lymphoid aggregates in lamina propria (H&E, 10x)

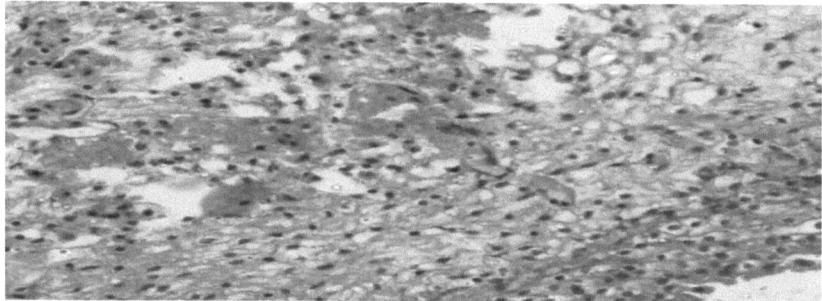

Figure -3: Chronic non-specific cystitis with lymphoid aggregates in lamina propria (H&E, 10x)

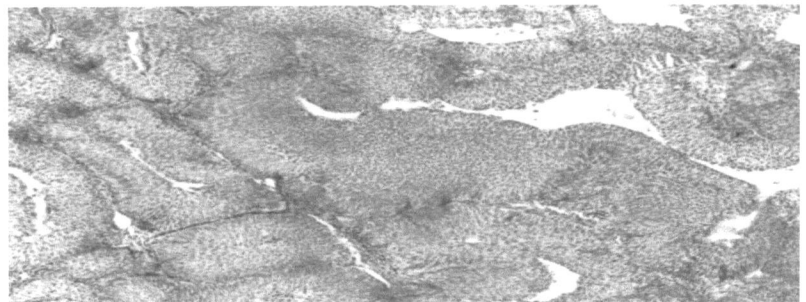

Figure 4: Papillary urothelial neoplasm of low malignant potential (H&E, 10x)

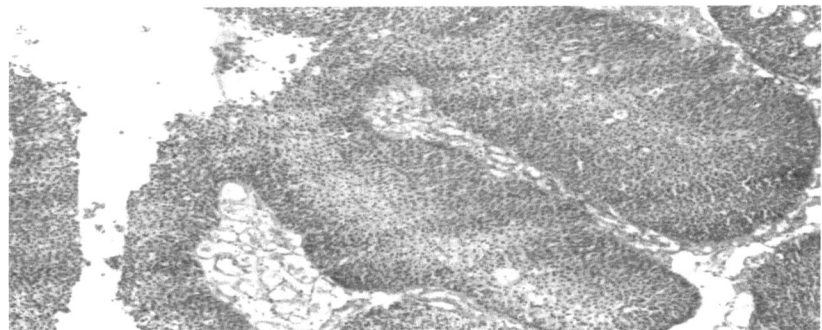

Figure 5 - Low grade papillary urothelial carcinoma showing papillae with mild pleomorphism of cells with maintained basal polarity (H&E, 10x).

4. DISCUSSION

The prevalence urinary bladder lesions in male cattle slaughtered at Debre zeit Abattoir was found to be 6.5% (21/325). In agreement with the current study, Herenda et al., (1990) from Canada and McKenzie (1978) from Australia have reported prevalence rates of 6.3% and 6.2% respectively. However, Sardon et al., (2005) in Spain recorded higher prevalence of 36.5% in bovine species. The higher prevalence rate in Spain has been mentioned to be due to the abundant presence of fern in the pasture which was incriminated as the cause of bovine enzootic hematuria and chronic cystitis.

Cystitis and cystic calculi with the reluctant cystitis have been the most frequently recognizes abnormalities of the urinary bladder of cattle (Blood and Radostits, 1994). In this study, macroscopic examinations of the urinary bladder revealed the presence of chronic cystitis and acute cystitis. Chronic cystitis (66.7%) was the most common lesion diagnosed although the cause was not identified. Herenda et al., (1990) and McKenzie(1978), have reported similar finding. In other studies elsewhere, the higher incidence of chronic cystitis (>60%) has been associated with bovine enzootic hematuria when cattle are exposed to grazing pasture contain bracken fern (peixoto et al., 2003). Clinical signs of acute cystitis were not detected during ante mortem examination but on postmortem examination of urinary bladder, lesions indicative of acute cystitis were observed. The higher prevalence rate of acute cystitis (33.3%, observed in this study was inconsistent with the report of Sardon et al., (2005) and Herenda et al., (1990).

I found the urothelial carcinoma was 86% out of total bladder carcinomas cases which were nearly correlated with the study of Eble and Young13 (80%) and Sharma et al., 14 (91.9%). Small no of cases of chronic non-specific cystitis was due to unawareness of symptoms by owner patient and biopsy was sent in most of the cases only for carcinoma by the veterinarian.

15

5. CONCLUSION AND RECOMMOENDATIONS

The lower urinary tract lesions in general and that of urinary bladder in particular are usually sporadic in occurrence. However, diseases of urinary tracts have considerable importance in many cattle raising countries. Problems associated with the urinary bladder can cause significant loss in the livestock industry particularly when they are complicated with obstructive lesions. Urethral obstruction presents an important economic repercussion for its ultimate prognosis following surgical intervention is often guarded. As this problem is basically a problem of male subjects, it results in decrement of much of the needed oxen power in potentially agricultural area. The current study has shown the prevalent nature of urinary bladder lesions in cattle slaughtered at this abattoir. The result showed the frequent occurrence of chronic cystitis. The role of chronic cystitis in causing urethral occlusion by tissue debris which resulted from chronic inflammation of the urinary bladder requires a due consideration in areas where urinary stones are not prevalent.

Therefore, based on the above given conclusions, the following recommendations are forwarded:

❖ Further studies should be conducted on causative agent's identification, histopathological study and risk factors of urinary bladder lesions so as to get clear picture about the urinary bladder problems.

6. REFE RENCES

Ayalew N. (2002): Preliminary study on prevalence of urinary bladder lesion of cattle slaughtered at Adama Municipality Abattoir, Shoa. DVM thesis submitted to College of Veterinary Medicine and Agriculture, Addis Ababa University, Bishoftu, Ethiopia.

Blood, D.c, Radostitis, O.M. (1994). Veterinary Medicen: A text book of disease of Cattle, Sheep, Goats and Horses, Bailliere Tindal, London. Pp. 531-538.

Campo, D.c., Jarret, W.T.H., Barron, R., Onel, B.W. and Smith, K.T (1992). Association of bovine papiloma virus type 2 and bracken fern with bladder in cattle cancer research **52:** 6898-6904.

Central Statistical Agency (CSA) (2003): Ethiopia Agricultural Sample Enumeration report on livestock and farm implement part IV, Addis Ababa, Ethiopia. Pp 29-139.

De-Lanunta, A and Habel, R.E. 1986). Teeth: Applied Veterinary Anatomy. W.B. Saunders Company USA. Pp 4-16.

Dobereiner J., Tokarnea C.H. and Canella C.FC 1967. Ocorrencia da hematuria enzootica decarinomas epidermoides no tratoo digestive superior em bovines nobrasil. Pesq. Agropec, Bras., Ser. Vet., 2:48 + -504 Evans W.C., Evans E.T.R 7 Hughes L.E 1954. Studies on bracken poisoning in cattle part I. Brit. Vet. J. **110(8):** 298_306.

Ehnen.S.J. (1990). Congenital defects of the urinary tract. *American Veterinary Medical Association* 197: 249.

Heeschen W. 1959. Die Haematuria vesicalis bovine choronica Dtsch. Tierarzti. Wschr. 66(22): 622-626, (24): 678-682.

Herenda, D., Dukes, T.W., AND Feltmate, T.E (1990): An abattoir survey of urinary bladder lesion in cattle. *Canadian Veterinary Journal*, **31**: 515-518.

Hironol., AisoS., Yamaji T., Mori H., Yamada K., NiwaH., Ojika M., Wakamatsu K., Kigoshi H., Niiyama K and Uosakiy. (1984). Carcinogenicity in rats of ptaquiloside isolated from bracken. Genn.**75**: 833-836.

Jones, T.C., Hunt, R.D., and Kink, N.W. (1997): Veterinary Pathology. 6th Ed, Lippincott Williams and Wilkin, USA. Pp. 664-667.

Keranso, S. (2010): Google Global Map. https://www.google.et/searcmap of Bishoftu/. Accessed on 25 May, 2014.

Mekenzie, R.A. (1978): An abattoir survey of bovine urinary pathology. *Australian Veterinary Journal,* 54: 41-49.

Nicholson, M.J and Butterworth, M.H. (1986): A guide to body condition scoring of Zebu cattle, (ILCA, Addis Ababa, Ethiopia). Pp. 72-74).

Ord'onez, N.G. and Rossai, J. (1996): Urinary tract, kidney, renal pelvis, ureter, bladder and male urethra. Ackerman surgical pathology 8th Ed, in: Rossai, J. (Ed.), Mosby, St. Luis. Pp.1059-1220.

Pamucku, A.M., Price J.M. and Brayn. G.T (1976): Naturally occurring and bracken fern induced bovine bladder tumors. Clinical and morphological characterastics. *Veterinary pathology* **13**: 110-122.

Peixoto. P.V., Franca, T.N., Barros, C.S.L. and Tokarnia, C.H. (2000). Histophtological aspects of bovine enzootic hematuria in Brazil. Pesquisa Veternaria Brasilaria **23**: 65-81.

Rao. D.S.T. Joshi, H.C. Kumar, M. and Singh, G.K. (1990): Pathological studies on bracken fern indiuced haematuria in calves and rats. *Indian Journal of Animal Sciences*, **60**: 654-656.

Raoofi, A., Mardjanmehr, S.H., Bokaii, S., and Laleh, A.R. (2011): Frequency of urinary bladder lesions in sheep and goats in Gramsar district: abattoir study. *Journal of Veterinary Research*, **2**: 113-116.

Roman, T.A. (2000): Retrospective study on ruminant urethral obstruction in Debre-Zeit area, Ethiopia. *Revue Medicine Veterinaries,* **151**: 855-860.

Rosenberger G. & Heeschen W. (1960): Adlefarn (Pterisaquillina) die ursach sog. Stallrotes der Rinder (Halmaturia Vesicalise Bovies chronic) Dtsch. *Tierarzti Wschr.* **67(8):** 201-208).

Rosenberger G. (1965): Longere Aufnahme Von Adlefarn (Pterisaquillina) die ursache der chronischen vesikalen Haematuria des rindes, *Wiener Tierarzti Wschr.***52(5):** 451-421.

Sardon, D., Fuente, T., Calonge, E., Perez-Alenza, M.D., Castano. M., Dunner, S., and Pena., L.(2005): Immunohistochemical expression and molecular analysis of urinary bladder lesions in grazing adult cattle exposed to bracken fern. Journal of comparative pathology, 132: 195-201.

Sharma S, Nath P, Srivastava AN, Singh KM. Tumours of the male urogenital tract: A clinicopathologic study: J Indian Med Assoc; 1994; 92 (11): 357-60.

Shimeles A. (2008): preliminary study on prevalence of urinary bladder lesions of cattle slaughtered at Gondar Elfora Abattoir, Northern Ethiopia. DVM thesis submitted to college of Veterinary Medicine and Agriculture, Addis Ababa University, Bishoftu Ethiopia.

Tokarina C.H., Dobereiner J. & Piextoto P.V. (2000): Planto Toxicas. Do Brasil. Editora Helianthus, Rio de Janerio. 320p.

7. Annexes

1. Estimation of ages of animals using dentition (Incisors)

Years	Characteristic changes
1.5 – 2	I- 1 erupts
2 – 2.5	I -2 erupts
3	I- 3 erupts
3.4 – 4	I- 4 erupts
5	All incisors are in wear.
6	I- 1 is level, and neck has emerged from gum.
7	I -2 is level, and neck is visible,
8	I- 3 is level, and neck is visible I- 4 may be level
9	I- 4 is level, and neck is visible
10	Dental star is square in I-1 and in all teeth by 12 years
15	Teeth that have not fallen are reduced to small round pegs

De- Lahunta and Habel (1986).

	Papilloma	Neoplasm Of Low Malignant Potential	Low Grade Papillary Carcinoma	High Grade Papillary Carcinoma
Architecture				
Papillae	Delicate	Delicate; occasionally fused	Fused, branching, and delicate	Fused, branching, and delicate
Organization of cells	Identical to normal	Polarity identical to normal; any thickness; cohesive	Predominantly ordered, yet minimal crowding and minimal loss of polarity; any thickness; cohesive	Predominantly disordered with frequent loss of polarity; any thickness; often discohesive
Cytology				
Nuclear size	Identical to normal	May be uniformly enlarged	Enlarged with variation in size	Enlarged with variation in size
Nuclear shape	Identical to normal	Elongated, round-oval, uniform	Round–oval; slight variation in shape and contour	Moderate–marked pleomorphism
Nuclear chromatin	Fine	Fine	Mild variation within and between cells	Moderate–marked variation both within and between cells with hyperchromasia
Nucleoli	Absent	Absent to inconspicuous	Usually inconspicuous	Multiple prominent nucleoli may e present

Annex 2. Histological features used to classify urothelial papillary lesions according to WHO/ISUP (2004)

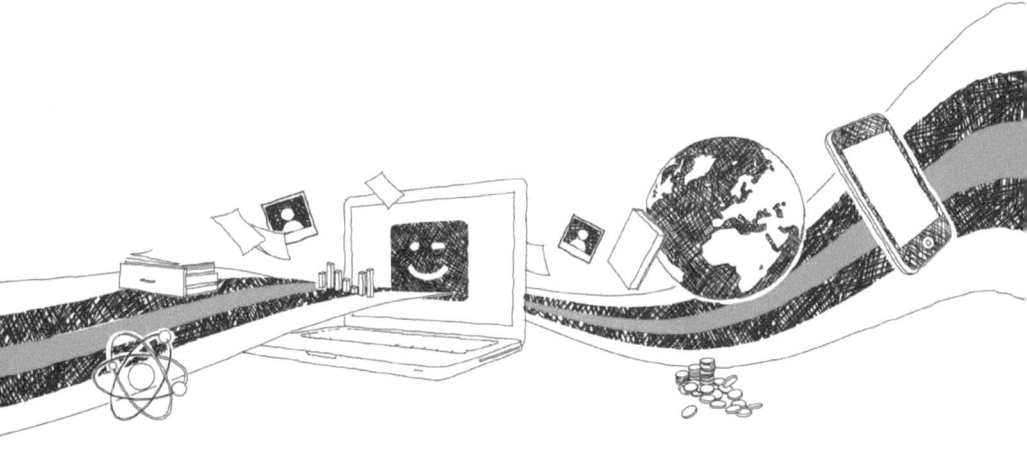
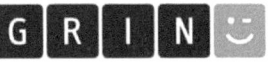